The Show Must Go On

Overcoming Obstacles Through Positive Thinking

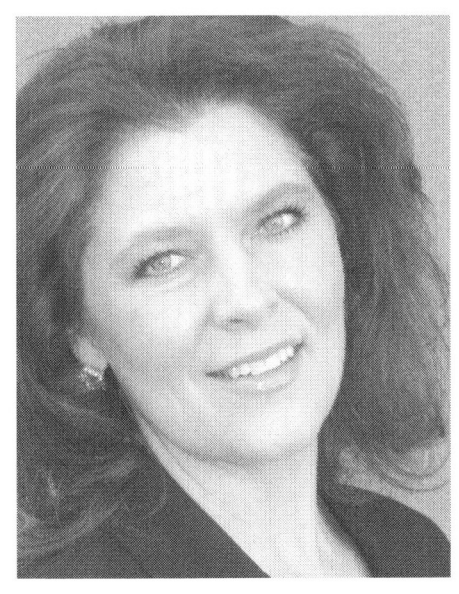

By Teresa Hill-Putnam

This book is dedicated to the people who have most inspired me:

- My three beautiful and very talented children, Ashley, Joshua, and Amber. I love each of you so much!

- My parents, Denis and Charlene Hill, who give me strength and encouragement.

- My dear childhood friend, Marcy Eastham. At the age of 12, Marcy died of heart failure. Although she was very sick and was waiting for a heart transplant, she never let her health problems get her down. I miss her so much!

- My lifelong friend, Penny Eastham, who had a heart transplant in 1985. She is a constant source of power and inspiration for me.

- All of my very special family, friends, and students. Thank you for being part of my life!

- Dr. Peter Quintero, for saving my life!

Contents:

4

Part One: My Story

Living With
A
Chronic
Disease

All About Me

My name is Teresa Hill-Putnam. I was born in 1970 to Denis and Charlene Hill. In 1999, I started getting very sick. I spent the entire year of 2000 in and out of the hospital. I was so sick that I was often unable to move, walk, roll over, sit up, or even feed myself. I had trouble breathing and was in respiratory failure when the doctors finally figured out what was wrong with me. In 2001, I was diagnosed with Myasthenia Gravis, a neuromuscular disease. Since then, I have learned some life changing lessons. I pray that my stories will be an inspiration to all that read them.

I am a single mother of three very beautiful, smart, and talented children. My children are what keep me going. They are what inspire me to get up each day, work hard, and enjoy the world around me. My children have been wonderful through my sickness and have learned to help whenever they are needed. Many times, it has not been easy for them.

My oldest daughter, Ashley (born in 1990), loves to dance and perform. She started dancing at the age of 2 years old. She dances/rehearses 25-40 hours each week, in addition to being a full-time student. She trains in ballet, tap, jazz, lyrical, and musical theatre. She graduated as Valedictorian for Tuacahn High School for the Performing Arts in 2009. She is currently a college student and is interested in Architectural Design, Dance, and Communications. She is a stellar student and is an absolute joy to me and our family. I don't know what I would ever do without her.

My son, Joshua (born in 1994), also loves to dance and perform. He is a very active and talented young man. He attends Tuacahn High School for the Performing Arts. He is an Actor, Singer, Dancer, and Performer. He is a good student in school and has a very fun and creative personality. He keeps our family smiling and laughing, even when times are tough. He helps me out a lot and is a wonderful young man!

My youngest daughter, Amber (born in 2004), is my little miracle! She loves to make us laugh and enjoys everything in life. Her sweet spirit gives us purpose. We certainly can't imagine life without her! After 7 years of desperately wanting another child, Amber was born. I was told that I would never have another baby because of my Myasthenia Gravis, but I proved them wrong. Amber is so much fun! She loves to sing, dance, play, and pretend. She keeps me young and gives me a reason to slow down and enjoy her world.

I appreciate my children tremendously! I know that we are strong because we love each other, we respect one another, and we work together as a team. We love the time we spend together and we've learned to support each other through every obstacle that life dishes out.

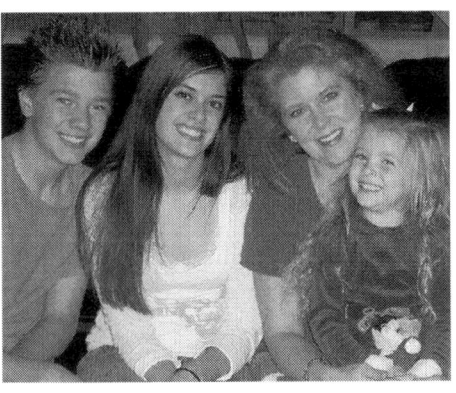

Josh, Ashley, Teresa, Amber

My Career

I started dancing in 1973, and have been teaching dance classes since 1984. I love teaching and directing ballet, jazz, tap, lyrical, Acro-gymnastics/tumbling, and musical theatre classes. I also enjoy writing scripts, directing musicals and performances for my students, and being a motivational speaker. Growing up as a dancer, I learned to take good care of my body. I have always been in very good physical condition. I try to eat a healthy diet. I don't smoke or drink alcohol, and I try to get plenty of sleep.

In 1994, I opened a Performing Arts School for Children in Littleton, Colorado called "Spotlight Performing Arts Center & Academy". After running the school for 12 very busy and successful years, I sold it to the Colorado Ballet and moved my family to Southern Utah. I now operate Spotlight Performing Arts Center, LLC in St. George, Utah. I enjoy teaching Dance, Tumbling, Acting, and Musical Theatre classes. I also direct the "Spotlight Performers" and "Spotlight Entertainers" Performing Companies and the "Ivins Children's Musical Theatre Company." As part of my services, I run a talent and booking agency for professional entertainers, Spotlight Talent and Entertainment. In addition to all of this, I offer motivational speaking seminars whenever I get the chance and I work professionally as a financial advisor on the side.

On a daily basis, I am very involved in the lives of my children and I enjoy volunteering at their schools. I love to dance, write, read, travel, and play with my family. I am thankful for all of the wonderful talents and opportunities that I have been given. I love sharing my story by speaking and teaching for large groups of people. I served on the Board of Directors for the Myasthenia Gravis Association of Colorado for several years, and plan to start a Myasthenia Gravis Association for Southern Utah as soon as I can. I enjoy people, and I strive to make a positive difference in the lives of others. My goal is to live each day to fulfill God's purposes for my life.

My Childhood

      I was born a month early because my mother had toxemia during the last stage of her pregnancy. I weighed 4 lbs 2 oz. I was put in an incubator for four days until I could maintain my own body heat. When I was eight days old, I was allowed to go home, with the stipulation that I have no visitors until I weighed six pounds. I was healthy except that when I cried, I could not catch my breath. By the age of 2 months old, when I cried I would pass out with the very first wail. The pediatrician started me on anti-seizure medication at 2 months old. The doctors ran many tests and said everything looked normal. Although I continued to be medicated, my episodes continued at the rate of 5-20 times per day.

      When I was about 13 months old, I weighed only 17 lbs and was not walking yet. One day, I went into a convulsion that the doctor could not bring me out of. After working on me for about two hours, I was transferred by ambulance to the University of Utah hospital, still in a semi-convulsive state. I was admitted for testing and observation. After two days of testing, the pediatric neurologist on my case informed my parents that I was a "breath-holder". He said that he thought my episodes at birth were uncontrollable, due to me being born prematurely, but that I had learned over time to hold my breath and make myself pass out to get attention. These "passing out" episodes often caused me to have seizures and convulsions.

The doctor also said that I had been so overdosed on my medication that he was surprised that I could even sit up. He reduced the amount of the medication I was taking, and I started walking within two days. He informed my parents that I would probably stop holding my breath if they tried to ignore it. The doctor advised my parents that when I had a seizure, they should put me on the floor where I would be safe, and walk out of the room. He recommended that they stay out of the room for at least one minute, but then to return to check on me. This way, I would learn that I did not get attention for holding my breath, but I would not be in any danger if I started to convulse and needed their help. Although difficult, my parents followed the doctor's recommendations and the daily episode rate of my seizures began to slow down.

When I was 20 months old, my father's job transferred my family to another state. Remarkably, out of nowhere, the breath-holding and seizure episodes stopped completely. I didn't have another episode until I was 25 months old, and my grandmother, aunt and baby cousin came to visit. Within thirty minutes of their arrival, I held my breath again. At this time, my parents realized how correct the doctor had been! My mother took me into the bedroom and scolded me. She put me on the floor, walked out, and shut the door. I never had another episode again.

At the age of two and a half years old, my parents enrolled me into ballet classes, hoping that I would become less accident prone and less rambunctious. Within one month into my ballet lessons, my parents saw a total turn-around. I became more motivated to excel and less interested in causing mischief. I learned to channel my hyperactivity into something productive. I even began to compete with everything my older brother, Rob, did. Rob is only 18 months older that I am. Even at a very young age, my motto was: "Whatever Rob can do, I can do better."— We were very competitive, yet we had fun. If Rob learned to do something, I had to learn it too. For example, when he learned how to tie his shoes to start Kindergarten…I learned how to tie my shoes within a day of him, at the age 3 years old.

I am a perfectionist and I am very competitive by nature.— Throughout my childhood, I tried to do everything *perfectly.* I was always at the top of my dance classes and academic classes, and I always received a lot of attention for my talents. I strived to be the prettiest, smartest, sweetest, and most talented child around.— I wanted to be perfect.

I did, however, push myself too hard. Until the age of 8 years old, I had many bouts with Strep Throat, but then I had my tonsils out and my Strep Throat episodes went away. As I got older, sometimes I did not take the time to eat enough and I often did not get enough sleep. When I was 10 years old, I got Mononucleosis-possibly from allowing myself to get so run down. I also had ulcers as a teenager. When I was 15 years old, I hurt my back, which put me into physical therapy for months. I worked hard in therapy and got back as quickly as I could. Although I had a few roadblocks along the way, I never let anything slow me down. I believe that this inner drive to succeed is the only reason that I am still alive today.

I was a concurrent high school student, attending high school classes in the morning and college classes in the afternoon. In addition to this, I danced at the University of Utah for 3-6 hours every evening and on Saturdays. Since I took most of my more difficult classes at the University, my high school experience was more for maintaining a social life than anything else. Hanging out with my friends was difficult with my busy schedule, but I found ways to MAKE THE TIME. I attended all of my high school dances and dating and parties were a big highlight of my teenage years. We did many fun and silly things in high school like barking at cars driving down the street, going cow tipping, playing "Truth or Dare", having massive snowball fights, going people watching, and just hanging out. Being a ballet dancer helped me learn to strive for excellence and be productive. My training also taught me how to take proper care of my body. I developed a great work ethic and a strong sense of discipline. At an early age, I learned to surround myself with morally healthy people. None of my friends drank alcohol, smoked, participated in illegal activities, or did drugs. I feel very fortunate that I never had to deal with the peer pressure involved in those activities. I had an insanely busy schedule during high school, but I had tons of fun. I managed to graduate from high school with a 4.0 GPA.

I got married right out of high school, one month before my 19th birthday. My husband and I were relatively happy for nine months and then I got pregnant. Everything went downhill from there. He was very controlling and abusive toward me during my pregnancy. Ten days after my new baby was born, I took my baby girl and fled to my parent's house in the middle of the night. We eventually got a divorce. I was only 20 years old.

I was determined that I would never marry again. I was scared to go on dates, but I had many friends. When I was 23 years old, my best friend asked me if I would marry him. He promised to take good care of me and my little girl. We got along very well and I liked the way he treated me. He was sweet with my baby and I believed that he would make us happy. I loved him very much as my friend, and I figured that I would grow to love him more and more as the years went on. We got married in September 1993.

I have always been strong physically and emotionally. As I have grown up, I have learned to take my stubborn streak, change it into determination, and channel it toward being successful. I learned to practice hard and to never give up. I was taught at a very young age that "The Show Must Go On!" Even when tired, sick, or upset, a professional dancer still has to go onstage when scheduled. This is a character trait that I have taken with me in all areas of my life.

I have always had tons of energy. Luckily, I am a focused, goal oriented and motivated person. I have known since I was a small child what I wanted to do when I grew up and where I wanted to go in life. I learned to direct my energy in positive ways through dance, school and performing. Even when I am tired or run-down, I am usually able to pull myself into action. I never let myself rest or have too much "down time." That is, until I got really sick and had no other choice...

**Enthusiasm is the greatest asset in the world. It beats money and power and influence.
It is no more or less than faith in action.**

-Henry Chester

Getting Sick

In1999, I started having episodes of weakness, especially in my arms, neck, and upper body. I also started having frequent headaches that I could not explain. Since I owned and operated a large performing arts school, I had to keep working and trying to act as if nothing was wrong. I was working about 60 hours a week and did not have time to be sick. I had to hire more help, and I often had to have my employees help me teach classes because I was too weak. Although I had been spotting the same Acro-Gymnastics students for the previous five years, I suddenly felt that I didn't have enough strength to hold their weight. I was worried that I was going to drop somebody. Assuming it was "just a phase" my body was going through, I didn't pay much attention to my symptoms. I knew I felt exhausted and figured that more rest was all I needed. I assumed my symptoms would eventually go away.

As time passed, I started coming home from work in the evenings more and more exhausted. I was out of breath all of the time, even when resting. Sometimes I was even too weak to speak. I would come home from work and go right to bed. I was usually too weak to eat dinner because I could not chew or swallow. I started coming home from work during the day to rest so that I could face my evening classes. When I didn't get to rest during the day, I was useless.

I didn't know what was wrong with me! I had always had so much energy! I hadn't changed my routine. I was eating the right foods. I was getting plenty of sleep. Why was I so wiped out? I am a dancer. I was used to being able to control every movement. I was very aware of my body, but was unable to make it do what I needed it to do. My brain would tell my legs to work, but they wouldn't. My neck was too weak to hold my head up. I could not put my arms above my head. My hands could not clench tightly enough to lift anything. Why couldn't I stand up from a chair or climb a flight of stairs without help? Why was I having trouble chewing, swallowing, talking and breathing? Something was definitely wrong.

My Struggle for a Diagnosis

When I started getting sick with Myasthenia Gravis, I went to see my doctor. I was having tremendous headaches and weakness in my neck, arms, hands, and legs. I was also having trouble eating and was always out of breath. My doctor told me that I needed to join a health club and start exercising more. The doctor felt this would help me reduce my stress level and give me something to do to pamper myself. The next day, I joined the local YMCA. I started by riding the stationary bike.

On my first day at the YMCA, I rode for about 5 minutes on the bike. I was exhausted and out of breath. I went home and stayed on the sofa for the rest of the day, unable to move. "Man," I thought, "I must be really out of shape!"

The next day was the same... After exercising, I was completely wiped out! Expecting to build up my endurance, I continued working out daily for the next few months. Instead of getting stronger, I was feeling weaker and weaker. My headaches worsened. The muscles in my arms, legs, and neck became even weaker. I felt like my body weighed a million pounds! I knew something was wrong with me, but I couldn't put my finger on it. Some days were better than others. Mornings were often better than evenings, and I usually felt better after a nap. I explained this to my doctor. She thought that my symptoms were being created by STRESS. Being a business owner, a working wife, and a mother of two children, I had a fair amount of stress- but not more than normal. I agreed to go see a psychologist.

After seeing the psychologist, I was sent back to my primary care doctor for another evaluation. The psychologist agreed that I had a high stress level because I owned and directed a Performing Arts School for nearly 700 children, but she was not convinced that my symptoms were caused ENTIRELY by stress. My primary care doctor sent me to see a different psychologist to get a second opinion.

The second psychologist suggested that I continue to reduce my stress level, and in the meantime, change primary care doctors. I took the advice and changed doctors to get the ball rolling again. My new doctor sent me to see a neurologist for evaluation concerning my increasing headaches and weakness.

The neurologist assumed that my headaches and sore neck *WERE* probably caused by stress and prescribed to me some medicine for migraines. I followed the directions of the neurologist, truly hoping for an answer and cure. I continued to get worse.

My headaches continued. My neck was weak and I had a hard time holding my head upright. My eyes were very tired, and my arms and legs were getting weaker. Walking wore me out. My stride was slow, and my left leg dragged. Stairs were becoming almost impossible. I was getting more and more out of breath with activity. My symptoms and severity were changing daily (sometimes hourly). Resting made me feel better, but with activity I would quickly get weak again. I knew that something was wrong with me, but my doctors didn't

understand. I started thinking I *was* crazy.
This is when I started getting ***REALLY*** sick!

As the days went on, I continued to get weaker. My husband and children (then, ages 9 years and 5 years old) started having to do everything for me. They had to take me to the bathroom, and help me walk up and down the stairs. They had to fix me meals, and bring me everything. Sometimes they even had to feed me. I was so weak that I couldn't even lift the utensil to my mouth. They had to do the dishes and clean the house. I had to stay on the recliner, because I was too weak to get in and out of my bed. I usually had to be propped up by pillows to help alleviate my troubled breathing and swallowing. I was often even too weak to hold up a book to read because I could not lift my arm to turn the page. Most of the time, rolling over was not possible. Resting did not seem to bring my strength back like it had before. I thought I was going to be paralyzed, and I truly was worried that I was going to die.

One day, I started having a heavy feeling in my chest. I was rushed to the hospital in an ambulance. I stayed in the hospital for several days, while the doctors ruled out heart problems. I didn't think the problems were being caused by my heart, but since I didn't know what was happening to me I agreed to get the tests run. I was sent home with instructions to return if I got worse.

A few days later, I was back in the emergency room. I was too weak to roll over or sit up without help. I couldn't swallow or feed myself. If I ate or drank anything, I would choke. My voice was weak and I was very short of breath. I could not hold anything because my fingers would not grip. The doctors decided to do an MRI on my brain. They ruled out Multiple Sclerosis and Stroke. They told me to make an appointment to see my primary care doctor the next day, and brought me in discharge papers to sign. I refused to sign discharge papers, and asked to see another doctor. I was NOT going to leave the hospital again until I had some answers. A Neurologist happened to be in the hospital, so he was brought in to evaluate me.

This Neurologist (I wish I remembered his name!) looked at me and asked me some questions. He left the room and came back with some interns and nurses. He explained that he wanted to give me a drug called Tensilon©. He said that he thought it might help me. He explained that he had not used the drug before, and that is why he wanted to have the other doctors and nurses in the room. Privately, he told my husband and parents that he thought that I might have Myasthenia Gravis. He explained that the drug, Tensilon©, was a test drug to help him determine a diagnosis. They decided that it was worth a try.

The doctor inserted the medicine into my IV and we waited. Almost immediately, I started to get remarkably stronger. I could sit up by myself! I could make a fist! I could hold a glass of water without dropping it! I could even stand up! I was strong again. I felt like I could run around the block! I was so excited that something finally worked!

The "high" lasted only about 10 minutes, and I started getting weak again. I was frantic! What was happening? Why did it stop working? I asked them to give me some more. Nobody had mentioned that Tensilon © would wear off so quickly. I thought it was a cure and I expected it to last forever. I was so disappointed! I asked if I could have some Tensilon© to take home. The doctor told me that Tensilon© didn't come in pill form, and that it was only to be given in a hospital. He told me that he couldn't prescribe any medication for me since he was an ER doctor and could not follow my case. He told me that the Tensilon© was a test that had worked exactly the way he had expected. He said that he thought I had a disease called Myasthenia Gravis, and to contact my Neurologist the following day for an appointment. I agreed and was discharged from the hospital.

Following my Tensilon© test, my HMO Neurologist couldn't get me in for an appointment for 3 weeks. I agreed to the appointment and waited. I continued to get weaker as the days went on. When it was finally time to see him in the office, he told me that he didn't actually believe the results of the Tensilon© test. He said that it worked because "I expected it to work". He said that he thought it was a "placebo effect". I could not believe it! The truth is, I had never even heard of **Tensilon ©** before. Only my husband and my parents were told what the drug was and what it might do. Nevertheless, I was at a dead end with this HMO neurologist. Looking back now, I think that this particular doctor didn't know enough about Myasthenia Gravis to treat me. Instead, he referred me to another psychologist. This time, I had had enough!

With the use of the Internet, I contacted the National Myasthenia Gravis Association. With their help, I found a neuromuscular specialist in SLC, Utah that worked with Myasthenia Gravis patients. I traveled to Salt Lake City to see him. He was very informative, and told me that I "probably had Myasthenia Gravis". He was not willing to run additional tests to make the positive diagnosis, however, or give me any medication because he was not able to follow my case so far away. He referred me to a neuromuscular specialist back in Colorado.

When I returned home from SLC, Utah, I contacted my HMO Company and asked for a referral to see this recommended neuromuscular specialist. Unfortunately, he was not covered by my insurance. They refused my request and told me to go back to the HMO Neurology office that I had been to before. Another dead-end!

I decided to call the recommended neuromuscular specialist's office in Colorado even though my HMO refused to pay for it. I decided that I would pay whatever it took to get my life back. The first appointment was six weeks away. I took it.

Six weeks later, I went to see the neuromuscular specialist. He told me that he couldn't follow my case, since he was not part of my insurance plan. He told me that he could "consult me" during the visit, but he would not run any tests, diagnose any condition, or prescribe any medications for me. He said that if my insurance changed, I could come back and see him. This doctor suggested that I "quit my job and go on disability" to see if I could reduce the stress level in my life and maybe I would get better. I told him to "go to hell", and left his office. I was fuming! Another dead-end because of incompetent doctors and restrictive medical insurance policies!

What was I to do? I wanted to be a Mommy. I wanted to run, dance, and skip. I wanted to hop in the rain puddles with my children. I wanted to travel. I wanted to go shopping. I wanted to run errands. I wanted to have enough strength to drive my own car. I wanted to pour my own milk on my cereal. I wanted to walk up the stairs by myself. I wanted to make dinner for my family. I wanted to go on a hike. I wanted to ride my bike. I wanted to go to the park and fly a kite. I wanted to go back to work to teach dance and tumbling classes, and run my Performing Arts School again. I eventually wanted to have another baby. I wanted to make my own choices. I wanted to be strong. I wanted to feel good. I wanted my life back!

I knew that there was something wrong with me, and I was DETERMINED to find an answer. I just couldn't understand why the Tensilon© test had made me feel so much better if it didn't determine anything! I knew that I had Myasthenia Gravis! I needed more answers, and I needed someone to listen to me...

Because I had no other choice, I decided to go back to my HMO doctor. I insisted that he give me an Acetylcholine Receptor Antibody blood test for Myasthenia Gravis. Hesitantly, he finally agreed to get the test done for me. I expected the test to come back positive. I expected to be able to show my doctors that I was right all along. I expected to *finally* be able to get the help I needed. I expected to get my life back!

Boy was I wrong! The blood test came back NEGATIVE. I couldn't believe it! After all of the research I had done on my own, I <u>knew</u> that I had Myasthenia Gravis. Plus, the Tensilon© test had worked. Negative? How was that possible? I couldn't believe it! Now what?

The HMO neurologist explained to me that the negative blood test *confirmed* that I did not have Myasthenia Gravis. (I have since found out that he was completely wrong about the blood test. At least 40% of all Myasthenia Gravis Patients have negative antibody tests.) He sent me back to the psychologist to help me deal with my stress level. I was out of answers, and I knew I needed someone to help me. Tail between my legs, I agreed to go…

Being a firm believer that therapy is an important ingredient to a healthy lifestyle, I didn't have any problem with going to see a psychologist. *My problem was, I knew something was physically wrong with me, but NOBODY was listening!* I was being told that my symptoms were all in my head. I was really starting to think I WAS crazy! The frustration I felt was enormous!

Nevertheless, I made an appointment with the referred therapist.

As I faithfully attended my therapy sessions, it became more and more apparent to me and the psychologist that something WAS physically wrong with me. I had a happy life, I was married (although, not always happily), I had two wonderful children, a nice house, and a job that I enjoyed. My physical symptoms and personal limitations were creating extreme anger, stress, and frustration, but I was psychologically sound. I had goals and dreams that I wanted to meet. My problem was, I had an inner drive that said, "go", but a body that couldn't move. As I got weaker and sicker, my therapist became more concerned.

A few days later, I ended up in the Emergency Room again. This time, I was having trouble breathing. The tests showed that I was getting enough oxygen, but the carbon dioxide level in my blood was too high. I was suffocating. My lungs were weak, and were struggling to work properly. The Emergency Room doctor put me on a high dose of Prednisone & Mestinon to help me get stronger. Since my body responded so well to the drugs, I was able to avoid being put on a respirator. The doctor suggested that I find new Neurologist immediately and get treated for Myasthenia Gravis.

I got home from the hospital, and called my friend from the Myasthenia Gravis Association of Colorado. She was very concerned about my condition. She made a few phone calls for me, and got me an emergency appointment that very day with her neurologist, Dr. Peter Quintero. This is the day my life began to change! After seeing Dr. Quintero, he had no doubt that I had Myasthenia Gravis. He ran the tests I needed to confirm a diagnosis. He was my lifesaver! I finally started getting the proper treatment that I needed.

The news that I had Myasthenia Gravis came with mixed emotions. On one hand, I was glad they had finally figured out what was wrong with me…but on the other hand, I was terrified because I had just been diagnosed with a chronic disease that I would have to live with for the rest of my life. I went through many emotions. Some days, I was sad and depressed because I felt sorry for myself and I felt very alone. Other days, I was happy and relieved that my disease was not diagnosed as something worse. Sometimes, I was scared and angry-all I wanted to do was yell and scream at everyone around me, because I needed to place the blame on someone or something for my pain. There were other times, that I was just glad to be alive.

Dr. Peter Quintero put me on a high dosage therapy of Prednisone (75 mg a day!). He also had me continue to take Mestinon every 2-4 hours, as I needed it to treat my symptoms. He had me come in to see him every week so he could monitor my progress and adjust my medications as needed. Dr. Quintero has even called me at home many times to make sure that I was doing okay. He treated me with kindness, dignity, and respect. None of my other doctors had done that. He trusted me to be smart enough to learn to manage my disease and not rely only on him.

Due to the high doses of Prednisone, I gained over 65 lbs. within just a few months, but I was finally able to breathe again. Although I was embarrassed about being fat, I decided that the weight gain was a small price to pay for the Prednisone saving my life. I started getting stronger and was able to return to some of the activities I had previously enjoyed. Although my activity level was still very limited by my lack of strength, I started going into work for a few hours every day, mostly to give me a purpose and to get me out of the house. I was finally able to drive again and I enjoyed spending time with my children. I was able to prepare some of our meals and sometimes even do a load of laundry.

Once I was strong enough, Dr. Quintero helped me to find a surgeon, and we scheduled my Thymectomy. Dr. Quintero monitored my care, and taught me how to adjust my medications and treatments as needed. Although he is retired now, I will never forget how much Dr. Peter Quintero changed my life! I have never met a doctor that genuinely cares so much about his patients. He understood that I wanted a better lifestyle, and was willing to do whatever it took to help me put my life back together. He believed in me. He encouraged me to learn about my disease so I could manage it and live a productive life. He helped me get my disease under control and he saved my life!

Ultimately… YOU are in charge of yourself. You know how you feel. Be your own advocate.

Listen to others, but don't let them control your life.

Patients must learn as much as they can about their disease. They must not only rely on their doctors (even specialists) to be the experts, especially if the disease is rare or uncommon. Patients must listen to their own bodies. They must find out about their own physical limitations and learn to work around them. Patients must fight for their right for good healthcare.

Never Give Up!

I have had to make some major changes in my life in order to feel well, but I am now doing better than ever! I firmly believe the saying, "The Show Must Go On!" So often, I see people giving-in to their limitations. Many of the people I have met who have Myasthenia Gravis and other chronic diseases have given up. Most of them have quit their jobs, and are on disability. It makes me very sad for them, because many patients do not believe that they can have a more normal life. Having Myasthenia Gravis myself, I understand that Myasthenia Gravis can be extremely difficult to live with. Some days are good; other days are horrible. I also understand that all cases of Myasthenia Gravis are very different. Some patients have Ocular MG (affecting only the strength in the eyes), and others have Generalized MG (affecting all parts of the body). There are also unlimited degrees of severity within the disease, and some symptoms are more severe than others. Nonetheless, patients must learn to live one day at a time. They must not give up on their dreams, sometimes they just need to find other ways to accomplish them. GIVING UP IS CERTAINLY NOT THE ANSWER!

In Feb 2000, my performing arts school in Colorado caught on fire. The smoke damage destroyed almost everything we had and left the building uninhabitable. Luckily, no one was hurt, but it was a terrifying and life changing experience! I had to get fifteen two and three year old little children out of the burning building, full of thick black smoke. I had nightmares for months following the incident. I thank God everyday for making sure that we all got out safely!

Being so sick at the time of the fire, I was tempted to give up and close my performing arts school. I decided that I could not do that. Instead, however, I decided to rent a temporary space in a nearby shopping center and move all of our classes there until our building could be fixed. I had students and employees who were counting on me, and I wasn't ready to give up on the business that I had worked so hard to build. Due to the fire and the move, over 50% of my students dropped. I also lost 3 employees during the 9 months that we were in the temporary space. Times were tough, financially and emotionally, but I pulled it off. We were finally able to move back into our building and start all over again.

After the fire, I felt like my children and my students needed and deserved something special. I took them on a Performance trip to Walt Disney World in March 2001. By this time, I was being treated for Myasthenia Gravis and I was doing a little better. Knowing that the trip could make me sicker, however, I decided to take some precautions. My doctor and I increased my medications for a few weeks before the trip, and until two weeks after the trip to give me some extra strength. Also, I rented a wheelchair when we got to Florida, so I could save my energy for the most important things. It would have been easier to stay home, but we would have missed out on the entire experience. The kids got to do several performances at Disney World and we took 26 rolls of film to help us remember how much fun we had! We loved riding on rides and playing together. I wouldn't trade this time for anything! It will be a trip we will remember forever!

My Challenges

In March 2001, I was started on high doses (75 mg/day) of Prednisone to make me stronger and prepare me for my Thymectomy surgery. The medicine made me gain over 65 lbs. It came on within about three weeks, and has taken years to get off. My weight has been a rollercoaster ride ever since, determined by how much Prednisone I am taking.

When my weight fluctuates, I sometimes get frustrated and I have to remind myself that it is only temporary. Without Prednisone, I would not be alive. A few pounds is a small price to pay for my life. I will continue to eat a healthy diet and exercise as much as I can. Because I will probably be on Prednisone for the rest of my life, this may be a never-ending struggle for me. I will make the best of it.

When I got strong enough from the Prednisone, I was able to have my Thymectomy surgery in June 2001. It was a life changing event for me. Your thymus gland is located next to your heart. It is a tiny gland usually about the size of a green pea that sometimes produces antibodies in Myasthenia Gravis patients that attack the body. Although it is not a cure, symptoms usually improve by removing the thymus. It is a major surgery that takes proper planning and many months of recovery. In order to get to my thymus, my chest had to be opened up- just like in open heart surgery. My sternum was split from the top of my chest to the bottom of my breastbone. My thymus was removed and sent to the lab for testing. My breast bone was wired back together and my chest was closed. My thymus it was found to be quite enlarged (bigger than the doctor's hand!), but luckily, it was not full of cancer.

When I woke up from the surgery, I had no idea how big the incision would be. The reality was devastating to me. My incision was much larger than I had imagined and I was all swollen up from the steroids that I was given during surgery. I was extremely upset. I had never felt so ugly! I knew from that moment on I would never be the same. For a long time, I covered up the massive scar on my chest and I refused to wear shirts that would show it.

Over time, however, I have learned that it doesn't really matter. Now, I wear whatever I want. My scar is part of me. It is a part of who I am. It is part of my past. It is a part of my journey. My Thymectomy surgery was well worth the pain, the scar, and the recovery. My symptoms have improved and I can now better manage my disease and live a normal life with less medication.

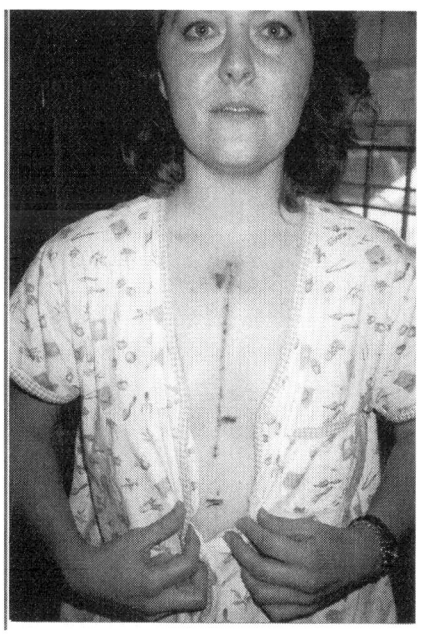

My Miracle

In October 2003, I received the best news ever. I was pregnant! Although it was not a planned pregnancy, it was MY MIRACLE! I had been told that I would probably not be able to have any more children, but I proved them wrong. Luckily, when I got pregnant, my health was stable and I was almost fully recovered from my Thymectomy surgery. The timing could not have been better! Pregnancy in Myasthenia Gravis patients is not well known. It is said, however, Myasthenia Gravis patients have a 33% chance of getting worse, 33% chance of getting better, and a 33% chance of having no change in symptoms while pregnant. I was a lucky one! Although my pregnancy was difficult, my problems were not caused by my Myasthenia Gravis. My Myasthenia Gravis symptoms actually improved during the pregnancy and I have been doing better ever since.

After spending 17 weeks on complete bed rest during my pregnancy due to many complications, I gave birth to a darling baby girl in April 2004.

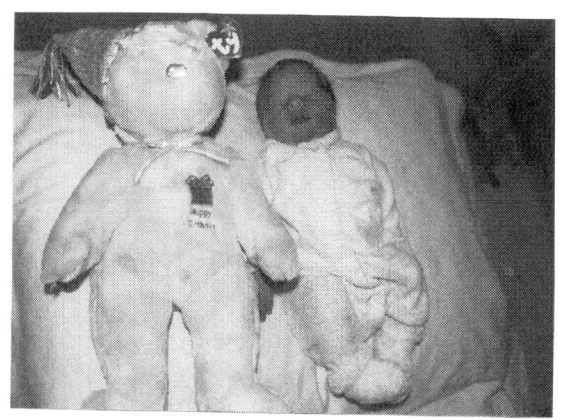

Amber was born two months early (at 32 weeks gestation), but was healthy and strong! She is such a blessing in all of our lives!

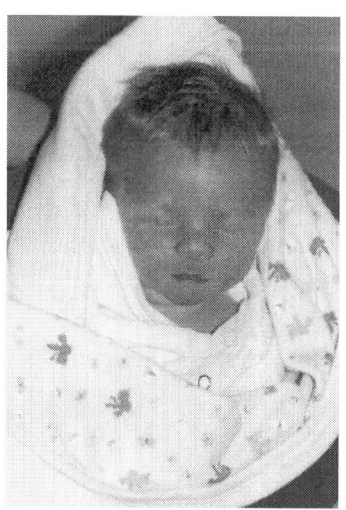

Big Changes

In August 2005, I sold my performing arts school in Colorado and I moved with my children to Southern Utah. I had been looking to move to a place with a lower altitude for several years. I chose St. George, Utah because of its mild winters, clean air, slower paced lifestyle, and natural beauty.

My husband stayed in Denver to work and sell the house. He did not agree with the move, as he did not see the importance of it. There was nothing I could do or say to make him understand. Since our marriage was rocky already, I decided that it wasn't about him anymore. I had to do what was best for me and for the kids, with or without his approval. I decided to take a chance and make the move, not knowing if he would ever join us in St. George or not. My daughter got accepted into a performing arts high school in St. George and we arrived the day before school started.

Just as expected, my health improved almost immediately when we got to

Southern Utah. We bought a house and got settled into our new community. The kids loved school and they had many opportunities to perform. I started teaching again and opened another performing arts school. We made lots of friends and were happy. Life was peaceful.

It took over a year for my husband to sell the house in Denver. Even after it sold, he didn't join us right away. He stayed in Denver and moved in with some of his friends. I think he liked being "single" and the freedom of having fewer responsibilities.

He finally decided to join us in St. George in January, 2007. Not sure what life would be like having him around again, I decided to give it a try. The entire year of 2007 is a big blur. After my husband joined us, my household became tense and unstable. He blamed me for everything, especially making us move to St. George. Although he was working, he refused to contribute much money to the household. He drank a lot and argued with me about everything. The kids hated being at home and so did I.

My husband had always been a drinker, but over time, he became more and more dependant on alcohol to help him deal with the stresses of everyday life. When I got sick, my husband turned to alcohol to help him deal with it. He never seemed terribly concerned about how sick I was, he just mostly complained about how my sickness would affect our income and lifestyle if I couldn't work. This made our problems much worse and made me feel more unloved and alone. Once I got physically strong enough, I told my husband that he could either stop drinking and get help, or I would divorce him. He refused to admit that he had a problem with alcohol and he chose divorce. Our marriage was over. I got divorced in March 2008, after being married for 15 years. I have no regrets.

When my marriage ended, I was left with a house that I could not sale for the amount that I owed, a huge mortgage that I could not afford, over $30,000 in personal credit card debt, and three children to raise...all with a chronic disease that I have to live with everyday. I felt angry, scared, and completely betrayed. I did not plan to marry an alcoholic. I did not plan to be a single parent with too many bills to pay. I did not plan to be stuck with a house that I could not afford. I certainly did not plan to get a divorce at age 38. I had some decisions to make-FAST! I had two choices, I could either let things fall apart or I could pull up my bootstraps and take some action. I had worked too hard in my life to let everything go. My children needed me to be strong and to provide stability for them again. I decided to take action.

I negotiated a loan modification with my mortgage company so that I could keep my family in our home. I opened a case with the Utah State Office of Recovery Services to review and collect child support and garnish wages. In addition to teaching and running my Performing Arts School, I decided that I needed to make some changes in my finances. A friend of mine sat down with me and helped me develop a plan to get out of debt, become properly protected, and to eventually be financially independent. I learned so much that I decided to become licensed to be a financial advisor part time. I am now licensed to help people with consolidation loans, mortgage refinances, and life insurance policies. I enjoy teaching my clients how to become financially independent. I am also currently training for my Securities license. I am on my way to a bright future and I am proud of all the hard work I have done to get there.

Living with Myasthenia Gravis has turned out to be much easier than I thought it would be when I was first diagnosed. Most days are good. All of the things that I have learned over the past 10 years outweigh all of the bad days I have had. I have learned to manage my disease to the point that most people don't even know that there is anything wrong with me. I have learned to listen to my body. I know exactly when to take my medication and how much medication I need to take. I have had to learn to pace myself and rest whenever I can. Working with children makes me happy, but it can be challenging because of all the germs they carry. Myasthenia Gravis is an autoimmune disease, which makes me more susceptible to sickness. Illnesses usually hit me more severely than most people, and it takes me a long time to recover when I do get sick. Because of this, I have to take extra precautions to stay well. I take a variety of vitamins everyday, I slather myself with lavender oil, and I wash my hands often. All in all, life is good!

There are NO problems in life that cannot be overcome.

My Spiritual Journey

For a long time after getting sick, I was VERY angry! I felt sorry for myself and could not understand WHY. I had been through so much already, and to find out that I had a disease that would never go away was a RUDE REALITY to have to face.

I was also angry with my husband, my friends, my family members, and my parents. As I saw it, nobody cared or understood me. They were all going about living their happy little lives, while I was sick, weak, and miserable! How could they entertain each other, laugh, and have fun? They didn't know how I was feeling. Did they not care? Why didn't they ask more questions? Why didn't they try harder to help me? Again, I felt so alone!

This is when I turned to God. "WHY?" I asked him. I didn't understand what I was supposed to learn from all of this. Why was my journey so difficult? I felt sorry for myself! I didn't understand why all of the people I loved seemed to become so cruel when I got sick. Why did they abandon me? Why didn't they understand me? Why didn't they care more? Why didn't they try harder to help me? Why did I feel so alone? Why did I feel so helpless? What was I supposed to do? Was I fighting this battle all by myself?

I felt like my entire world was caving in around me. For two years prior to my getting sick, I had been begging my husband (who is now my ex-husband), to let us have another baby. He said that he absolutely did not want to have any more children and wouldn't even talk with me about it. This was a huge problem in our marriage. Then, when I was at the weakest time of my sickness, on New Years Eve 2000, my husband asked me if I would be okay with him donating his sperm to his lesbian friends so that he could father a baby for them. I could not believe it! I had begged and begged for another child and he refused! He wouldn't give a baby to his wife, yet he was willing to give a baby to his friends? This was a hard hit for me! This was the beginning of the end of our marriage. My very own husband was throwing away our relationship at the weakest and sickest time in my life. How could he do this? I was hurt and angry. I felt betrayed. I knew at that very moment that I needed to get well, for the sake of myself and my children. This blow could have done me in, but I knew I could not give up. This gave me an even bigger drive to seek the help I needed and get strong again. I turned to God for help.

After many months of deep thought, depression, tears, and prayer, my answers started coming together. Unlike I had previously thought, I was not all alone, God was with me. He had been with me all along, but I was not looking for Him. I had been so angry that I was not seeking God's presence in my life. He was the only one that could really understand the emotions I felt inside. He was the only one who could provide the comfort I needed. He was the only one who could give me strength. He was the only one who could successfully help me fight this battle and win.

God helped me to understand that most of the people around me DID care. Although they didn't completely know what I was going through, they were TRYING to help. I was frustrated because I was expecting others to make me strong and well again. When I couldn't fix my problems myself, I was unfairly expecting others to fix them. Sickness and disease make many people uncomfortable. Sickness also can make patients feel frustrated and angry. Often times, people don't know how to respond, and they come across as if they don't care. Many of my friends and family members were waiting for me to ask them for help when I needed it. Many did not know what to do or how to help. Many did not want to offend me by offering their services. Many chose to ignore the fact that I was sick. Somehow they thought that I might get well if they ignored my symptoms. Some made no contact with me at all.

God helped me to realize that even though people do the best they can, they are human. He also helped me to understand that I cannot expect people to be perfect. He helped me to see the goodness around me. He helped me to realize that I was not alone.

I believe that one of the reasons I got sick was to bring me to a closer relationship with God and appreciate life at a whole new level. When I am well, I have a tendency to be very independent and rely only on myself for everything. I used to believe that "if you want something done right, you must do it yourself." I have learned so much since I got sick. I have learned to ask for help when I need it. I have learned to rely on God to help me. "Soar on wings like eagles; run and not grow weary; walk and not be faint." (Isaiah 40: 31) I look to God when I am tired and weak. I have learned to surrender my worries to Him, and rely on Him to hold me up and make me strong. Since I have learned this, he has never let me down. I have a sense of peace now. I am no longer scared or angry. I know that with God's help, there is nothing I cannot handle. I believe that God has an important purpose for me. Part of my purpose is learning to live with Myasthenia Gravis, and sharing what I have learned with others. I am very blessed.

"I can do everything through Him who gives me strength." (Philippians 4:13)

Do Genetics Play a Role?

I don't know if my Myasthenia Gravis has genetically played a role in the health and development of my children. Only time will tell, because so much is still not known about the disease and the genetic factors.

Although all of my pregnancies were very difficult, my children are worth every effort. I had severe morning sickness with each pregnancy, and suffered premature labor with all of my children. They were all born early and were premature babies.

Ashley was born 6 weeks early, but was the healthiest of all my children. I spent 14 weeks on complete Bed Rest with Joshua and he cost us over $100,000 before he was even born. Joshua was born at 33 weeks gestation. I spent 17 weeks on complete Bed Rest with Amber, and I was only able to get out of bed to use the restroom. She was born at 32 weeks gestation. From birth, all of my children struggled with apnea, as do many premature babies. They would stop breathing and turn blue, mostly when they were eating or sleeping. These episodes would sometimes happen 30 to 40 times per day. Although very frightening, we had to remind them to breathe until their little bodies and brains could learn to maintain breathing on their own. They each were on Heart Rate/Apnea Monitors until they were about 2 years old. Thankfully, they all eventually outgrew their apnea problems. All of my children are healthy now, but all have had some bumps along the way…

Ashley was a very shy and timid child. She has suffered from extreme anxiety and has had to learn to become more confident in social situations. Ashley got ear infections, colds, flu, pneumonia, and strep just like other children, but she has never had to deal with anything serious. Ashley has Asthma and uses an inhaler when exercising. During the past year, she has developed some stomach problems - probably due to stress.

Joshua has had respiratory problems since birth. His lungs were weak when he was born, and he got RSV at three months old. Throughout his childhood, Josh has suffered from dozens of bouts with

Pneumonia and was diagnosed with Asthma when he was 3 years old. He had to have weekly allergy injections for several years to help minimize his allergy triggers and asthma symptoms. We are very lucky to have his breathing and allergies under good control at this time. He has learned to be smart about his asthma and make adjustments in his life as needed. Josh also has ADHD, which could stem from being a premature baby. I have taught him to channel his energy in positive directions like dancing, singing, tumbling, and acting. He understands his talents and his limitations, and he doesn't let anything stop him.

Although Amber was born at just 32 weeks of pregnancy, the nurses told us that she was "small but mighty." They were right! Amber, however, started having seizures at the age of 7 months and she was eventually diagnosed with Epilepsy. I am not sure if her seizures have anything to do with the seizures I had as a child, or if it is just a coincidence. She takes anti-seizure medication several times a day, plus we also have an emergency medication that we can use if she has a severe seizure that gets out of control. We have to take extra precautions with Amber and watch her more carefully, but instead of making these health problems run her life, we are trying to give her a sense of normalcy. She doesn't know anything different.

I pray that as my children get older, they will have strong and healthy lives. Often, autoimmune diseases tend to run in families, and I hope that my Myasthenia Gravis has not been passed to them. If so, we will deal with it. I feel very lucky to have such wonderful, talented, and supportive children. I would not trade them for the world!

"Dear Lord, Please give me…
The patience to listen.
The courage to speak.
The honor to follow.
The wisdom to lead."

-Unknown

"My Mommy Has Myasthenia Gravis"

by Ashley Putnam

This following story was written by my daughter, Ashley, at the age of 12 years old. It was published in 2002 by the Myasthenia Gravis Association of Colorado, as a children's picture booklet to help children and adults gain a better understanding of Myasthenia Gravis. We had it Copyrighted in 2003.

My mom has a disease called Myasthenia Gravis (MG). Sometimes it is quite hard for me to understand. Mommy says that her body is like a TV antenna that doesn't work correctly. Her brain sends the right signals to her nerves, but her muscles do not always respond.

Sometimes when my mom wakes up in the morning, she feels great and we can play all day. Other days, she has no strength at all, and she can hardly get off of the sofa. When my mom first got sick, I was very scared. Her arms and legs were weak, and she could hardly sit up or roll over by herself. Sometimes, Mom even had trouble breathing and swallowing.

The doctors did not know what was wrong with her, and I was worried that I was going to get sick, too. Once the doctors figured out what was wrong with Mommy, they explained to me that Myasthenia Gravis is not a contagious disease. The doctors do not know what caused Mommy to get sick. They also do not know how to cure Myasthenia Gravis, but they know how to treat it using surgery and medicines.

I have had to learn to help Mommy more since she became sick. Sometimes I have to help take care of her. It has taken me awhile to understand that Myasthenia Gravis doesn't just go away. Sometimes I feel angry that Mommy is sick.

Last summer, my mom had to have surgery as part of her treatments. The doctor took out her Thymus Gland (in her chest by her heart). It took a long time for Mommy to heal after her surgery, but she is doing much better now. You see, Mommy's Thymus Gland was making chemicals called Antibodies that were attacking her body and making her muscles not get the right signals from her brain. Since her surgery, Mommy feels much better.

Mommy has to take medicine every day to help treat her symptoms and make her muscles work better. The medicines she takes every day are called Mestinon and Prednisone. These medicines help to make Mommy strong. Now Mommy can dance, run, and play with me again!

Josh's Story

By Joshua Putnam

This story was written by my son, Joshua Putnam in 2003, when he was 9 years old.

My name is Joshua Putnam. My mom started getting sick when I was 5 years old. I was in Pre-School. I remember my mom and me taking a "quiet time" together everyday while we read and watched "kid" movies. Often, my mom didn't feel very well and she was tired all of the time. I didn't mind reading and watching movies with my mom, but I sometimes wanted to go to the park or ride my bike. Since she was sick, my mom didn't always have the energy to do this with me. Sometimes, this made me mad.

Since I have Asthma, I understand what it is like to be sick a lot. I have had to learn to take good care of myself so that I don't get sick as often and so I don't make my mom sick. When I was a kid, I had to get allergy shots every week. I seem to be getting better as I get older, so I am lucky. I wish my mom could outgrow her sickness, too.

Over the years, I have had to learn a lot about Myasthenia Gravis. I know that it makes people weak. I also know that it can make people have a hard time breathing and swallowing. When my mom gets sick, I have to help her more. I sometimes have to even help her go up and down the stairs. I help her carry things. I sometimes have to do extra chores to help around the house. I have had to become more responsible than most of my friends. Sometimes I think it is not fair, but then I remember all of the things my mom does for me.

Even though my mom is sick, she tries to stay active and do as much as she can. She still runs her Performing Arts School, and she takes us to perform at lots of fun places. We sometimes get to travel to perform, too. Some of our Performance Trips include: Disneyland, Disney World, a cruise to Mexico, Mt. Rushmore, Las Vegas, and San Antonio.

My mom always tries to help us have fun and learn a lot. She is involved in my school and activities. She also takes good care of me. I appreciate all of the hard work and fun the things that my mom does for me. Even though she has Myasthenia Gravis, she doesn't let anything stop her. I love my mom and respect her a lot. She is a great example for all of us.

Part 2:

Words
of
Wisdom

Throw yourself a Pity Party, but Set A Timer!

Every person feels sorry for himself once in a while. It is normal to feel angry, frustrated, or sad when faced with a problem, chronic illness, a major life change, or a difficult situation. It is very important to learn to deal and cope with these feelings. It is also very important to learn how to look past the negative aspects of life, and focus on the positive.

Every morning, I spend about 30 minutes by myself. I spend this time thinking, reading, praying, and planning my day. Sometimes, when I am having a bad day or when I am not feeling well, this time is spent feeling sorry for myself. When I feel helpless, sad, depressed, angry, or frustrated, these feelings seem to take over all of my thoughts. One very helpful thing that I have learned to do is to throw myself a "Pity Party."

I know that I need to allow myself time to feel and work through these negative feelings. The trick is to not let them ruin my entire day. **This is when I set a timer.** If I give myself a specific amount of time to feel sorry for myself, I can acknowledge the feelings I have and start dealing with them. When the timer goes off, my "Pity Party" is over for the day, and I have to move on. This routine works great for me. You may want to give it a try, too.

Pull up your bootstraps and keep on going. Turn Lemons into Lemonade.

Some days are just going to be difficult. If you expect those days to happen occasionally, you will be ready for anything that comes your way. Don't let anything throw you off balance. Make it a game. As with everything, PRACTICE MAKES PROGRESS. If you practice making good things come out of bad situations, you will learn to be good at it. Think of a bad situation and make up a good ending. Not only will this help make you a good problem solver, but it will also help make you more optimistic. I sometimes play this game with my little girl.

This is the way we play the game:
        I might say, "What would you do if you missed the school bus?"

My little girl might reply, "I would come home and we would have a tea party together."

I might say, "What would happen if you fell off the monkey bars?"

She might reply, "I would get back up and try it again."

I might say, "What if you broke your arm?"

She might reply, "A cast would make it all better."

I might say, "What if we get lost on our way to Disneyland?"

She might reply, "At least we'd be lost together."

The responses don't have to be actual solutions, just ideas. The more you play the game, the more fun it becomes. And… it can prepare you for the difficult times in real life.

**Learn to appreciate how lucky you are and count your blessings.
When you feel down and out, do something nice for someone else.**

Hug the people you love and remember to say, "I Love You!"

Life can change in an instant.
You never know when you, or those
you love, will be gone forever.

Live each day as if it were your last.
Live each day as if your loved ones
will be gone at midnight.

Cherish the moments you share with
others.
Make each moment count.

Treat others the way you want to be treated.

Do something nice for someone everyday.

Never underestimate the power of a kind word or good deed.

Look for opportunities to make others feel important.

Respect and appreciate others.

Be grateful and acknowledge those who have helped you.

Never forget where you came from.

Remember that no one makes it alone.

Give others a positive reason to remember you. What will your legacy be? How will you be remembered?

Relax and Breathe...

"Life is not measured by the breaths you take, but by the moments that take your breath away."

-Unknown

Take time to smell the flowers... and enjoy looking at the stars.

Notice even the smallest details in your life.

Have you ever seen a painting by Thomas Kinkade? He is an amazing artist who is known for his paintings of landscapes and cottages. His work is much different than any other artist I have ever seen. His paintings contain all of the little details that most people never even notice—detailed blossoms and leaves on every tree, tiny pebble stones on the walkways, individual bricks on the houses, snowflakes, and tiny feathers on every bird. He doesn't stop there, though. Thomas Kinkade is called the "Painter of Light". With his tiny paint brush, he is able to capture the essence of real light within his paintings. The detail is amazing. When I take time to enjoy his work, I am reminded of how many little details in my own life I am overlooking. The beauty we have been given is spectacular. Take time to see it.

Everything we do in life can become a new learning experience to keep growing.

If people stop learning, they die.
Find something to learn in every life experience…

Even boring routine things (like doing laundry) can be rewarding if you find something to learn each time you do it.

Find the lesson to be learned in your experiences and take pride knowing that you are learning something new.

Leave the world a little better than you found it.

This will give you purpose and add more excitement to your life.

USE your talents or you will LOSE them.

Learn everything you can and strive to be all that you are capable of.

Look for new opportunities to grow and learn.

People in your life are there for a reason.

People are in your life for one of
two reasons. Either they need to
teach you something, or they need
to learn something from you.
Make your relationships rewarding
and meaningful.

Stop blaming others.

Take responsibility for your
own actions.

Don't hold grudges and
try to be forgiving.

Remember that we are ALL human.

Be the first to admit when you are
wrong and apologize if necessary.

Everyone Makes Mistakes.

Learn to forgive others and move forward. If you do not, you will create a miserable life for yourself. Eventually, you may have no one left on your side.

Be careful not to be too critical.

Never "close a door" or "burn a bridge."

"To forgive is the highest, most beautiful form of love. In return, you will receive untold peace and happiness."

–Dr. Robert Muller

Learn to listen.

Often times, people and opportunity knock softly.

It takes time and effort to become a good listener, but it is well worth it.

If you miss what people are trying to tell you, you may miss out all together.

Make a "To Do" List everyday.

Make a list of things you need and want to do. Cross items off the list when they are completed. This will make you be more productive in life. It will also let you see how successful you really are.

Take control of your life.

Simplify your home and be organized.

Slow down…
Take time to enjoy the people and the
things that really matter.

Manage your time wisely.
Don't procrastinate.

Run your own life…
Be careful not to let your life run you.

Take time to balance your life and your time.

WORK
8 hours
each day.

When you are at work, work hard.

When you get off of work, stop
working.

Always be on time.
Time that is lost can not be retrieved.

SLEEP
8 hours
each day.

Take a 20 minute "Power Nap" each day if needed to rejuvenate.

Monitor the amount of sleep you get each night and make it a priority.

Keep a notepad by your bed.
If you wake with a good idea, write it down.

LIVE
8 hours
each day.

Do something nice for yourself
everyday.

Plan and enjoy vacations.

Eat out and enjoy the company of
others.

Spend time outdoors.
Enjoy the beauty of nature.

Dare to be Different.

Let people know what you stand for
and stick to it.

Actions speak louder than words.

Be a good example.

ALL
OF THE
WORLD
IS A STAGE.

You may never get a second chance to make a first impression.

Be positive and enthusiastic.

Enjoy Life.
It is not a dress rehearsal.

Always be honest and truthful.

Live each day with purpose.

Do something important everyday.

Live each day as if it were your last.

Make your life count.

Think BIG thoughts.

Dream BIG dreams.

Set short-term and long-term goals.
Be the best you can be.

Work to meet your true potential.

> "It is time to start living the life you've imagined."

-Henry James

Take the time to recognize and enjoy your achievements.

Judge your success by the peace, health, love, and joy around you.

Strive to make a difference and work to inspire others.

"Who you are is God's gift to you…

…What you become is your gift to God."

-Unknown

Take the time for Daily Exercise

When I was so sick, I was very frustrated that I could not exercise. If I sat on the floor, I could not get up without help. I was used to dancing everyday, and being very physically fit. I really enjoyed exercising, especially taking dance classes! The more physical activity I had when I was sick, however, the weaker I became. I came to the conclusion that I probably would not be able to participate in high-impact aerobics classes or dance classes anymore, so I needed to find another way. I looked into many different exercise programs, and decided to try Pilates. I have learned to use a ball to exercise with, and even on my worst days, I can now exercise lying in my bed. I modify my routine daily based on what I can physically handle. Some days I am able to do more than other days. Nevertheless, I can still exercise! Even just a few minutes a day of exercise makes me feel more energized.

Smile!

You never know, your smile may be the only one that someone gets all day.

A simple smile can change the world!

"When life's problems seem overwhelming, look around and see what other people are coping with. You may consider yourself fortunate."

-Ann Landers

Be
HELPFUL
to others.

"When a friend is in trouble, don't annoy him by asking if there is anything you can do. Think up something appropriate and do it."

-E.W. Howe

Enjoy being at home.

Make your home a place of sanctuary for
you and your family.

Make it a comfortable and peaceful place
that you will enjoy day after day.

Make your home a place where others will
want to gather with you
for fun and sharing.

"Success is the ability to go from one failure to another with no loss of enthusiasm."

-Winston Churchill

"Change your thoughts and change your world."

-Norman Vincent Peale

"Never worry about numbers. Help one person at a time, and always start with the person nearest you."

-Mother Teresa

"One hundred years from now, it will not matter what kind of house I lived in, what kind of clothes I wore, or how much money I had...
but the world may be different because I was IMPORTANT in the life of a child."

-Unknown

"It is our attitude at the beginning of a difficult task which, more than anything else, will affect its successful outcome."

-William James

"Dance like nobody is watching.
Love like you will never get hurt.
Sing like nobody is listening.
Dream like Heaven is on Earth.
Perform from the Heart!"

-Unknown

**"Every day
brings a chance
for you to
draw in a breath,
kick off your
shoes, and
DANCE."**

-Oprah Winfrey

"A man can get discouraged many times, but he is not a failure until he begins to blame somebody else and stops trying."

-John Burroughs

"Even if you are on the right track, you will get run over if you just sit there."

-Will Rogers

"When you are following your energy and doing what you want all the time, the distinction between work and play dissolves."

-Shakti Gawain

Take the time to do what you love.

Everything happens for a reason.

Try to find **GOOD** in everything.

Many people have reported that they would have never looked for their current job, if they had not lost their last one.

Sometimes we do not understand why things happen, but remember:
"When God closes a door…
He opens a window."

"Adversity is another way to measure the greatness of individuals. I have never had a crisis that didn't make me stronger."

-Lou Holtz

Try, Try, and Try again!

"Believe that there are no limits but the sky."

-Unknown

"Obstacles don't have to stop you. If you run into a wall, don't turn around and give up. Figure out how to climb it, go through it, or work around it."

-Michael Jordan

"Success seems to be largely a matter of hanging on after others have let go."

-William Feather

Keep journals, scrapbooks, and photo albums.

Everyday before I go to bed, I open my journal and write down what I am most thankful for that day.
Sometimes it is a simple sentence… At other times, I write an entire page.

I keep all of my important papers in a scrapbook. These things include: playbills from shows my children perform in, special drawings that my kids make just for me, report cards, certificates of achievement, awards, letters from friends, etc.

I photograph all of our important events and keep them chronologically in photo albums. I don't pick up the film from the store until I have time to go straight home and put them in an album.

My photo albums create wonderful memories for me and my family.

If you are not part of the solution, then you are part of the problem.

Would you agree that some people just like to complain?

I think that people should not be allowed to complain about things, without being able to offer a solution to the problem.

If more people tried to help find solutions, the world would be a better place.

Life is good.
Celebrate it!

Enjoy the world around you.
Acknowledge the beauty.
Smell the roses.
Gaze at the stars.
Hug your children.
Cherish and appreciate your spouse.
Do something nice for others.
Pamper yourself.
Praise and worship God.
Be creative.
Write a story.
Pet your dog.
Learn to LOVE your life.

"Energy is the essence of life. Every day you decide how you're going to use it by knowing what you want and what it takes to reach that goal, and by maintaining focus."

-Oprah Winfrey

FUN
IS WHAT
YOU MAKE
IT!

Create some fun for yourself,
every single day of your life.

"You must take personal responsibility. You cannot change the circumstances, the seasons, or the wind, but you can change yourself."

-Jim Rohn

"Strength does not come from winning. Your struggles develop your strength. When you go through hardships and decide not to surrender, that is strength."

-Author Unknown

Believe in yourself!

Be brave and take calculated risks.

Figure out what you want in life
and make it happen.

"If you LOVE the life you live…
you will live a life of LOVE."

-Unknown

When all else fails… EAT CHOCOLATE!

It always seems to perk me up
and it makes me feel much better!

.

24203147R00072

Made in the USA
Charleston, SC
15 November 2013